With A Little Help From My Friends

Elizabeth Fleming

ISBN-13:
978-1492170945

ISBN-10:
1492170941

Dedicated to my family, for all their love and understanding

the story of Elizabeth Fleming
in her own words

When Elizabeth Fleming was born in difficult circumstance, it was decided that she was dead. She was taken to the mortuary. It was only when the doctor when to certify her death that he noticed a tiny movement.

This is the inspiring story of a life that almost didn't happen, a life spent overcoming the difficulties caused by Cerebral Palsy and by people's reactions to disability.

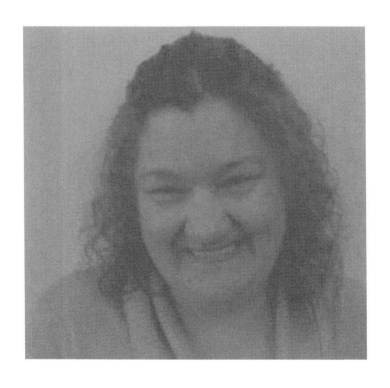

I often thought of writing about my life and the difficulties my family and I have had to face. There was no one around to ask how my disability would affect things. I felt bitter against the world.

Why me? Why not somebody else?

You know, if I had the chance to go back now, I wouldn't change a thing. I'd like to take out my bad parts, but no one's perfect. I've always known that I'm very lucky to have had such a loving family and such very good friends and I'd like to thank them for all they've done to shape me into who I am today.

With A Little Help From My Friends

Chapter 1

I was born on 21st December, 1966. When my mum arrived at the hospital she was met by a nurse. The family doctor had not arrived by then. It was a new doctor in the practice and this was going to be his first delivery. My mum told me that there was a great panic and the nurse knew Baby (me) was in distress, but didn't know what to do. As my mum delivered me, the cord was tangled round my neck and this was preventing me from breathing properly. The nurse ran for help. All of a sudden, there were people everywhere. They tried to revive me by putting me in hot and cold water. They just forgot about my mum. They couldn't revive me and they went back and told Mum she had given birth to a baby girl, but that she had only lived for fifty-five minutes. By now the doctor had arrived and asked to see me. I had been placed in the hospital mortuary. The doctor noticed one of my eyes flicker. "This child is still alive," he said. I was then transferred to the main hospital in Edinburgh under a police escort. The police contacted my dad and told him of my arrival and my demise in the middle of the night.

At the Western General Hospital I was put in an oxygen tent. As I had been starved of oxygen for so long the doctors knew I would have some form of brain damage, though how severe no one knew. By the time my dad arrived at the hospital, he was still under the impression that I had died, so it was a shock for him when my mum told him I was still alive, although I was still very ill.

The hospital suggested to my mum and dad that it would be a good idea to have me Christened, just in case I didn't make it.

My name still hadn't been chosen.

Dad said I should be called Flora after his sister and my mum agreed. At the time, my Auntie Flora's husband, George, was ill, so my Auntie said they shouldn't use her name as it might be bad luck.

It was then decided that my name should be Elizabeth, after my mum. Funnily enough, my condition improved as soon as my name was changed. My Uncle George sadly died soon after this.

My mum was allowed to go home three days later as it was Christmas time and she had my two older sisters, Diane and Moira, to look after. The hospital advised my parents not to come and see me as they did not think I would survive. My dad, however, visited me on Christmas Day. When he saw me, he prayed that I would live especially as I looked so much like him. After that, my mum visited every day to feed and bathe me. At 6 weeks old, I was finally allowed home.

On the day I arrived home, my big sister, Diane, can remember me being carried in a yellow carry cot. Diane was seven years old and Moira was four-and-a-half. At this time I had to be kept at the same room temperature. For a whole year my mum and dad took in turns to sit up at night and keep my room at an even temperature. I had to be taken to hospital three times a week for a check-up. My mum had to take two buses to make the journey to hospital as we had no car at the time. The doctors never gave my parents much hope and always told them I would never be able to do anything for myself. How wrong they were!

*

One day my dad was at work and my mum was at home with me and I sat for the first time. Mum was so excited and pleased with me she jumped on the bus to Musselburgh and took me to my nana's. No one believed my mum as it was several weeks before I decided to do it again. From then on, everything I managed to do was a great achievement.

At the hospital they said I would never smile or show emotion and it would be most probable that I wouldn't even recognise my mum from my dad. When the family were told the bit about me not going to smile, they all laughed because I am not one for smiling a lot.

There was a time that if my mum put anything around my neck, I used to go into hysterics. My mum couldn't understand this, but when she told the doctor he explained that it must have been caused by the trauma of my birth.

As I progressed, the doctors said it would always take me longer to do things and this has been very true.

At two and a half years old I still could not walk. I used to roll everywhere. Even when I was potty trained I used to roll to my potty. I slid on my bottom down 14 stairs with my sisters who made it into a game. I had not control of the muscles in my face and used

to slaver all the time, but my family helped
me to control this.

*

At three and a half years, my parents were
advised to take me to a playgroup. When
Diane and Moira were small there weren't
any playgroups. My mum took me every
day, but I cried and did not like it. She hated
to leave me, but once she'd gone I'd settle
down. My mum says she was sorry she had
to make me go as she feels I was too young.

Being the youngest of the family meant I
was very spoiled and was used to getting
everything my own way. It must have been
hard for Diane and Moira. Moira used to
feel left out as I needed so much attention.
Diane was older and very mature for her
age, so she didn't notice so much.

I always wanted a bike when I was little. Mum and Dad refused to get me one as I didn't have good balance and could easily fall and hurt myself. Being the determined person I am, I insisted that it was the only thing I wanted, so they eventually gave in. My first bike had three wheels, two at the back and one at the front. I had the time of my life riding around on it.

Chapter 2

When I was older, I attended a clinic in Edinburgh for people with disabilities. They gave my parents some hope. At the hospital, they always said I would never achieve anything, but at the clinic they said positive things. Looking back I recall how nervous I was for every visit. Mum never told me where we were going until the day beforehand. If I'd known in advance, I'd have had nightmares. I knew they were nice people and didn't intend to hurt me, but when anything was out of my normal routine I got very upset. I have had many different doctors and therapists and I know they were there to help, but it often got to be too much for me and my family. I often think it would have been better if there hadn't been so many people involved.

When I was five-and-a-half years old I started school. Up until then, I'd never walked far. I wouldn't go in a buggy either, so my dad had to carry me on his back. I took a furry toy in with me and had my photo taken with another girl from my class.

My first teacher was Mrs S. I can barely picture her.

School was very difficult for me as children can be very cruel to each-other. They realised I was different from them and so they made fun of me and called me names. One day I was upset and asked my mum why I was different from the others. She told me that I was very special and that God had made me this way for a reason.

Up until then, I suppose I must have thought that I was the same as everyone else.

Growing up in a normal world is hard for anyone, but having a disability makes it even harder.

Mum thinks that if I'd gone to a school for disabled people that life would have turned out differently.

It was difficult being the bottom of my class at everything.

I knew lots of answers for things, but because I couldn't write them down quickly enough, so knowing answers didn't count.

In Primary 2, my teacher was Mrs B. She was a lovely person. I was chosen to be an angel in the Christmas Nativity play. Mum came to watch me, but couldn't see me through the tears. I wore a white sheet and a silver halo. I was so excited and it's something I'll never forget.

In Primary Three there was a remedial teacher who helped children with difficulties. She was very nice. There were three of us who used to go together. I did now feel then that I was different from the others.

The Primary School was near the Infant School. This made the change much easier for me when it came.

Classes were split into four.

My teacher was very strict. Going from a small school to a big one was difficult. There were far more children to make fun of me. By then I was fed up with being teased, so I started to fight back.

Even though my family kept telling me that 'sticks and stones will break my bones, but names will never hurt me', I found it hard to keep to and unfortunately fought back.

They called me 'Jelly Legs' and 'Mongol'.

At parents' evening, the teachers said that I didn't try at school. All previous teachers had been impressed by my effort and understood that it was difficult for me.

Primary Five came and went.

My Granny Fleming died that year, but I was very young and did not really understand it. We moved house and as usual I did not like the change. I cried all the way to the new house. It was 5th November and there were bonfires everywhere. The house had just been built and as it was at the top end of town, it seemed too far away.

Mum and Dad had wanted to move because the place had so many bad memories. The new house had a very happy feel to it. My new friend from school moved in three doors away from me.

Ann, Mary and I used to play together. The new house was really good and we all settled in well.

Primary Six was a very good year for me. My new teacher was Mrs L. She was very kind to me and helped me to improve in so many ways. Up until then, I'd not been able to hold a pencil properly, but Mrs L helped me to manage this. Next door to us in

Primary Six there was a male teacher called
Mr B. He was a very nice person. He was
looking for children to play in the basketball
team. I was never much good at sports, but I
decided to give it a go. He picked all the
best players for the A-team, but there was
also a B-team and I was chosen to be in this.
I was so excited to get home and tell my
family. I went to all the training which was
after school. I was never any good, but Mr
B and the rest of the team encouraged me all
the way.

When I got a shot at the basket, which
wasn't very often, they all used to cheer. It
was great to be part of a team. Having
Cerebral Palsy sometimes made me feel
very lonely. I know people thought because
I walked and spoke differently that I had no
feelings, but I did. Mostly I kept the bad
things to myself, though, because I knew
that the things that were said to me hurt
them just as much as they did me.

I was asked if I would go swimming with a group of disabled people. I did not go because I did not feel I was like them. I used to feel bad for not going, but I went swimming with the mainstream school and loved it.

Mrs L left to have a baby half-way through the year. I missed her because she'd always been on my side.

As Christmas drew near, our PE class was allowed to do dancing. I was never picked because the boys said I slavered too much. At the party that year, there were lots of people who felt left out. Mr B came over and asked me to dance. I was so happy. He was so kind. I often wonder if he knew just how happy he'd made me.

In Primary Seven, my teacher was Mrs S. It was our last year of Primary School.

The police came to give us our Cycling Proficiency Test. We had to take our bikes to school. It was great fun because I loved my bike. I passed my test and it was a great achievement. When I went for my yearly check-up at the clinic, they were very pleased with my progress and said I wouldn't need to go back again. This was good news as I had never really got used to going. You would have thought that it would get easier over the years, but it never did.

Before leaving Primary Seven we had to put on a show. I was Mickey Mouse. I must have looked very funny with my big ears and black nose. This was a brave thing for me to do, to stand up in front of an audience. I guess I must have been a lot more confident back then.

Chapter 3

Going to Secondary School was a nightmare for me and for my family.

On the first day we all gathered in the main hall. We were split into different classes. We were told at Primary School we would be separated and moved into classes, but they assured us that one or two of our friends would be in our class.

All the names were called except for mine and my friend, Ann's. We thought this meant we would be in the same class. Then Ann's name was called and I was left in the hall with 10 other children. I didn't know any of them. Three of them were girls and seven were boys. We were taken to a small room where an elderly lady with white hair spoke to us. It felt strange in the small room with the other children. In my old class there had been thirty of us.

The lady's name was Mrs S. She said we were her children and she would take care of us. I asked to go to the toilet, but instead I ran home. This was the start of the worst experience of my life.

Mum and Dad were really surprised when I arrived home as I had been really looking forward to going that morning. They took me straight back, but I did not stay. I did not go to school for three months. I was taken to several doctors to find out what was wrong with me. Everyone gave different advice. I hated seeing all my friends going to school every day without me. I was so miserable and I was breaking the hearts of my family. I would never like anyone to go through what I did at that time. Eventually the lady from my old clinic asked if I'd go to school if Ann was with me. I agreed.

It made things better, but it was still very difficult. I had missed so much that it was virtually impossible for me to catch up. Once I had settled in, I met a very nice teacher called Mrs M who became a good friend. Mrs S and I had never really got on as it felt like she wanted to take over my life. She told Mum once that she could have made something of me, and she may have been right, but she made me feel so different to everyone else and that's something I never wanted to be.

Mrs M, on the other hand, treated me like everyone else. She was a very gentle and friendly person. She had a very sweet voice and if you did things wrong, you received a telling off that would mean it was dealt with. She was never angry with me for very long and I know I must have driven her mad sometimes. I used to tell her I couldn't do things and she'd tell me that if I thought about it I'd be able to. She was right about that.

Mrs M became my guidance teacher.

When I was choosing my subjects in third year, she told my mum that she'd never let me have her best china to carry but that she'd give me her daughter to look after and that she was far more precious than all of her dishes put together. My mum explained that this was a lovely compliment.

Mrs M and I still exchange Christmas cards and when me meet we always have a good old natter about the old days.

I was never one to enjoy going on holiday. As I've mentioned, I didn't like changes in life. We went to Butlins four times, but I didn't like it there because it was too busy.

I did like going to my Auntie and Uncle's farm in Aberdeenshire. It was so peaceful and my Auntie Elma used to take me fishing in the burn on the farm.

In 1980, Mum's brother was to celebrate his 25th wedding anniversary. Auntie Thelma and Uncle Martin invited me to go down with them and my nana. They lived in Devon, so it was a long way. We decided to go as Nana was getting old and she had four grandchildren and one great-grandchild she had never seen. I really wanted to go because had never met my cousins who lived there.

Mum, Dad, Nana and I got into the car and off we went. It was an eighteen hour drive. Nana and I slept most of the way. My dad was exhausted from the drive and slept for two days when we arrived.

I had such a great time and didn't want to return home as there was so much to do.

My uncle worked at the naval college and we all went for a sail there. It was lovely and I enjoyed the silver wedding and the company and meeting all the relatives.

When I was fifteen, my sister Diane got married. Moira and I were bridesmaids. I had never been to a wedding before, so I was very excited. Mum bought three outfits and six hats before she finally decided what to wear. She hadn't worn a hat for many years.

Dad wore a kilt. He looked really smart.

When he tried it on for the first time, though, his fat stomach was sticking out and we all laughed. He stormed out of the room, but we apologised and he felt better.

On the day of the wedding the sun was shining. In the morning we went to the hairdresser's to get out hair done. She made us look lovely. Moira decided we should go out for a drink. We were late getting back and Mum and Dad had been worrying about where we were. We just had time to get ready.

All our relatives arrived and the house was full of people.

Diane was a beautiful bride. Everyone told my parents that they must be very proud of their three lovely daughters.

The street outside our house was full of friends and neighbours. We felt so happy that day.

*

At the church Mrs M and Irene were there to see us. Irene and John were invited to the reception and it was really nice to see them there. I felt fine and when the music began and we walked down the aisle, I was shaking. Moira held on to my arm and I made it to the end.

It was a lovely service. We knew the minister very well.

The meal at the reception was lovely. I say beside the groom's dad. John's mum and dad are really nice. John is like the big brother I never had. Everyone had a wonderful time. Ann was my partner as we danced the night away.

Chapter 4

At sixteen, it was time for me to leave
school and get a job. I left with 3 GCSEs in
History, Modern Studies and Nursing
Studies. I knew it would not be easy to get
work as there are so many things I find very
difficult. My main ambition was to work
with young children. Mrs M thought I might
go to college and study for a Nursery Nurse
course. This frightened me, though, and was
the only time Mrs M showed how angry she
was with me. I was so upset at her being
angry, but she was only trying to help. I was
very self-conscious then and had no
confidence in myself. Mrs M knew me letter
than I knew myself. She phoned my mum
that night. The next day, we met and both
laughed and I apologised for being such a
wimp.

Mrs M had a sister who worked in a nursery
in Prestonpans. She asked the boss if I could

go and work there. It was a Parents' Evening when I first went to meet them. As I entered the gate, my heart was pounding, but I carried on. My first impression was that everything looked so tiny. Then a small lady came over and introduced herself. She told me her name was Mrs W and that she was very pleased to meet me. We had a look around and I met the other two ladies, Mrs D and Mrs C. Mrs W asked me if I would go in for a day and that was all it took to frighten me, so I ran away. Mrs M was not in the least surprised. I thought I had spoiled my chances, but Mrs M took me home and told me to sleep on it, which is what I did. Just by chance, a girl I knew was going to work at the Nursery on work-experience, so I went with her.

The children came in and they all looked very nice. The morning went very quickly. The ladies were all lovely and friendly. Mrs W asked me if I would like to go along for another day and I told her that I'd love to.

And that's how it all began. It was suggested that I worked for one day at a time on a voluntary basis.

At sixteen-and-a-half, I did not feel ready to go out into the working world. I felt so young and insecure and I kept thinking about school. I only worked for a few days a week at the nursery. Slowly I began to put in more hours and before I knew it I was going there on a daily basis and stopped thinking about the past. My sister, Moira, married seven months after Diane, so the house felt really lonely. It was hard for us to adjust to there only being three of us left. Mrs M came to see me and I told her I'd always be grateful to her for introducing me to the nursery and for giving me the chance to work with so many nice children and people.

In August 1984, my sister Diane had a baby. This was great for both families as he was the first grandchild on either side. Diane had Ross at 10:30 in the evening, so we didn't see him until the next day. I was full of great joy I got from seeing him. He was a very happy and contented child and I enjoyed taking him out for walks in his pram. He seemed to grow very quickly and he was walking at nine months old. In June 1985 we all went to the gala. Ross was dressed in a red outfit and we were all very proud. After the gala, we all went home to party f or my dad's birthday.

In July, my favourite Auntie, Auntie Jean was taken to hospital after suffering a stroke. My Uncle David came to tell us and it was a nasty shock for everyone. That evening, Mum and I went to see her and she looked very pale and tired. I cried when I left the hospital.

Auntie Jean slowly got worse and three weeks later she died.

This left a great space in my heart as I truly loved her. I regret that I didn't ever really tell her that. Now I like to think of all the good times we had together.

Chapter 5

Dad worked as a miner from the age of
fourteen.

At the age of fifty he was offered the chance
of early retirement and he took it.

With his redundancy money he and I
decided to start our own business selling
cosmetics and toiletries, so in November of
1985 I left the nursery.

Dad and I went to the warehouse and bought
lots of things to sell on. We sold them on
Saturday and Sunday mornings.

Soon after that, Mum had a heart attack. She
was taken to the hospital where Auntie Jean
had died. This made me afraid to go and
visit her. In the end, I went with my sister
Diane. I was relieved to see that Mum
looked fine, though she was still on a heart
monitor.

She eventually came home and needed a lot of rest.

Nana, who still had her house, was finding it hard to cope with things when Mum couldn't help her anymore. It was decided that Nana should go into Eskgreen Nursing Home in Musselburgh.

Mum felt guilty about having to make this decision, but it was for the best. Things like this make you realise just how much you can take your parents for granted.

Now it was my turn to look after Mum instead of the other way around.

Moira, married and living in Port Seton, made Christmas dinner for us all that year.

Mum's health slowly improved and in about a year she had fully recovered.

In May 1987, Diane had a baby girl, Nicola Elizabeth. She looked just like my dad and me when she was born. She now looks like her gran and her Auntie Moira. Moira's baby girl was born in October. She called her Julie. Julie had a mop of red hear just like her father. Ross was now the big boy even though he was only twenty-months old.

As the toiletry business never really got off the ground, I now found myself unemployed. I started feeling really unwell. I wasn't suffering from pain, just a lousy feeling which wouldn't go away. Mum sent for the doctor and he gave me tablets and telling me that my illness would soon pass. Things didn't get better though. I had no way of explaining how I was feeling and my mum got me to see another doctor, who diagnosed me with depression. I'd been getting really nervous about doctors because of my experiences. Dr B was very kind to me and this helped me to get to trust her.

She felt my depression was due to the death of Auntie Jean and my mother's illness. It also might have had something to do with me not having a job.

She suggested I contacted Mrs W at the nursery to find out if I could possibly go back there to work.

Mrs W agreed.

I was apprehensive at first, but my confidence soon came back. All the staff and children were very welcoming and I soon settled back into working life. My depression soon lifted and getting through it helped me to grow up. With Mrs W's understanding, I once more overcame my difficulties. I realised what good friends these people were for me.

Chapter 6

My family and friends.

DAD

Dad is a very kind and loving man. His hobbies are fishing and dog racing. We have a good relationship. His weakness is that he never thinks he's wrong. When the horses are on TV we always have a little flutter. If my horse wins, he says it was the one he was going to choose. I have only ever had one big win. I won £90 once and I gave everyone a little of the money. If Dad wins, he buys something for Mum and I. Dad thinks that he is the boss, but really it's my mum who has the last word. He has a very happy nature and he makes us all laugh by telling us stories about his younger days. One thing we all have in common as a family is that we all like to talk.

MUM

Mum is the most important person in my life. She is a caring person and always gives me good advice. I think she must feel smothered by us all because we all want to be with her all the time. I fell I can tell her all my problems and she is my best friend. Her bad points are that she is grumpy in the mornings and she always likes the house to be very clean and tidy. If I win the lottery, I will buy her a new fitted kitchen. I like to go shopping with her especially for new clothes (she has such good taste).

Sometimes we argue, but we don't fall out for long. Mum and Dad have a hard time caring for all of us, but I know they are proud of us all and I am grateful for all they have done.

DIANE

Diane is seven years older than me.
Sometimes I look on her as a second mother.
I always feel very secure with her. She has a
very strong character. She has a quite nature,
but can be short-tempered. She was always
very clever and she studied hard. Her life is
busy with two children to look after and she
works in a bank.

MOIRA

Moira is a very happy-go-lucky person.
She's always full of fun. She's firm with her
daughters, but they are very good children.
She likes to go out and sing at Karaoke
nights. Life hasn't always been kind to her.
Her marriage broke down, but she's a
survivor and she eventually met someone
else. Derek is her fiancé and he also has a
little girl. They all live together as one
family. Moira and I have become closer in
the past few years. I love having two sisters
and would certainly be lost without either of
them.

ROSS

As Ross was the first grandchild, there was great excitement leading up to his birth. He was always a very happy baby and rarely cried. He has grown up very quickly and he is now ten years old. He has a very gentle and loving nature, although he is a typical boy who likes to climb trees and gets up to lots of mischief. I doubt if he would deliberately hurt anyone's feelings. I think because he is the only boy in the family I tend to spoil him. We have a very special relationship. I used to worry that people made fun of him because of me being the way I am. One day I was reading the first part of this story to Mum and didn't realise the children were listening in. Ross asked what it was like when I was in the mortuary. Whether it was cold. He wasn't pleased when everyone laughed. Because I could never pronounce my name properly, Ross has always called me Auntie Bibby and I really like to hear him say it like that.

NICOLA

Nicky was born twenty-one months after Ross. She wasn't as contented a baby, but it was soon discovered she had a bowel complaint which made her irritable. Nicky will be eight this year and she is quite a girl. She has lots of confidence and talks all the time.

JULIE

Julie is really quiet. She was born five months after Nicky. Julie's mum and dad separated when she was only three. Before the separation she was a very clingy child, but she has grown into a lovely child. She goes to her dad's at the weekends and lives with her mum all week. Moira and Dennis both have new partners and Julie now has a little sister.

KIRSTY

Kirsty came into our family two years ago at the age of three. At first she was very shy, but she was young enough to adopt. Julie was really kind and shared everything with her. She has become part of our lives. She and her dad, Derek, have made Moira very happy.

MY FRIENDS

As I was growing up, I really only had two special friends, Mary and Ann.

Ann was in my class from day one of the first school. Ann's dad and my dad also grew up together.

We had other friends as well. Ann left school six months earlier than me and we drifted apart for a while. I invited her to my twenty-first party and this brought us together again.

She's married now and has a wee girl called Ann-Marie and she is due to have another baby soon.

Mary and I first met at Primary School. She was clever and an all-round athlete. In some ways Mary was everything I would have liked to have been. When we moved in to our new home, Mary lived three doors away. Mary's mum worked so her dad took her to all the sports meetings. Sadly, her dad died when she was only ten. After that, Mary's mum and auntie used to go and see him compete. The most memorable event was when she went to Meadowbank stadium to watch her run in a four-hundred metres race. I watched her from the stand with her mum and auntie. Mary ran the race of her life and won easily. The race was televised and we must have watched the video of it a hundred times when we got home.

When I became claustrophobic, I had to stop going to the running track. That made me sad because I really enjoyed going. Mary and I are still good friends and our families are also very friendly. We sometimes have them over for supper. We have a good time talking. Marys Auntie Mary died last year and we all miss her very much.

I met Irene at my first school. She was a teacher and she lived around the corner from me. When she walked her dog, Shane, I asked her if I could go along and that was how our friendship began. I always seem to get on with people who are either older or younger they seem to understand my difficulties easier than people my own age. I can confide in Irene and trust her. If things go wrong for me, I like to know that she is there and ready to listen.

I first met Leona at the Nursery eight years ago. I had just started and she gave me a lift to and from work. We used to have good chats. She is a very quiet and refined person and we got on very well. When she stopped coming to the nursery with Joanne, we lost touch for a while. I started helping at the Brownies and when Joanne joined the Brownies we met up again. When Diane had Nicki, Leone also had one called Gemma. Leona helped me through my depression as she is a good listener and a good friend. Her husband took us to Brownies and I had one or two panic attacks in the car, but they were both very understanding. I really appreciate people who understand my difficulties. Although I have given up helping at Brownies, we have remained friends.

Chapter 7

Ross came to Mrs W's nursery when he was three. He settled really well and I was proud of him. He spent a year with us before going to school nursery. He didn't' like school much and I think it was because I wasn't there. Julie also came to the nursery and it was lovely having her around. Mora went back to work and Julie went straight to the school nursery. Moira had split up with her husband at this point, but the whole family coped well.

We used to go to Musselburgh every Saturday to visit Nana in the nursing home. Nana always had sweets.

One Saturday, Diane and I went along with the three little ones. Nicky asked for a sweet and she chose a Murray Mint. It was too big for her and she choked. Diane lifted her and ran screaming for help. The matron took Nicky and put her fingers down her throat. In doing so, she managed to push the sweet down the whole way. Nicky started to cry. It was the sweetest sound I'd ever heard. Matron had saved her life.

Ross, Nicky, Julie and Kirsty all accept me for who I am. They have never known me as anything else and as they grow up, I hope they will still see me that way. The ladies at work have said they'll help me write this story down and I hope it will help people to understand what life is like for me and for others like me.

I've omitted some parts, the most difficult times, as it's too difficult to face them just now. Maybe I'll get to those one day.

My depressions made life feel impossible at times. I'm now on medication and this helps. I also need to take control of myself.

At twenty-eight years old, I'm still the subject of name calling. Only the other evening, as I was locking up my moped, some young lads went by and shouted at me. I'd done nothing to deserve it. It makes me feel like I'm being punished. If only they knew how much it upsets me, maybe they'd leave me alone.

I'd like to thank everyone for helping me to grow into the person I am today. Being disabled has brought many problems, but I've never ever been short of love. Thanks to all concerned for the happiness I've had until now.

-end-

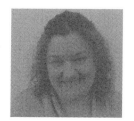

Printed in Great Britain
by Amazon